ELHEM JBEBLI

DIBASIC PROTEIN INTOLERANCE

ELHEM JBEBLI

DIBASIC PROTEIN INTOLERANCE

Straddling the metabolic and autoimmune divides

ScienciaScripts

Imprint
Any brand names and product names mentioned in this book are subject to trademark, brand or patent protection and are trademarks or registered trademarks of their respective holders. The use of brand names, product names, common names, trade names, product descriptions etc. even without a particular marking in this work is in no way to be construed to mean that such names may be regarded as unrestricted in respect of trademark and brand protection legislation and could thus be used by anyone.

Cover image: www.ingimage.com

This book is a translation from the original published under ISBN 978-620-6-71438-5.

Publisher:
Sciencia Scripts
is a trademark of
Dodo Books Indian Ocean Ltd. and OmniScriptum S.R.L publishing group

120 High Road, East Finchley, London, N2 9ED, United Kingdom
Str. Armeneasca 28/1, office 1, Chisinau MD-2012, Republic of Moldova, Europe
Printed at: see last page
ISBN: 978-620-7-69918-6

TABLE OF CONTENTS

I. INTRODUCTION

Dibasic protein intolerance or protein intolerance with lysinuria (LPI) (OMIM #222700) is an autosomal recessive inherited metabolic disorder. It is linked to a defect in the membrane transport of the dibasic amino acids Arginine (Arg), Ornithine (Orn) and Lysine (Lys) caused by a mutation in the SLC7A7 gene encoding the y + LAT-1 subunit of the transmembrane transporter of dibasic amino acids. This transporter is expressed in the basolateral membrane of the renal tubule, intestinal cells, the lung, the spleen and in circulating monocytes and macrophages, which would explain the broad spectrum of symptoms described, These include growth retardation, protein intolerance, hepatosplenomegaly, osteoporosis, pulmonary involvement, renal failure, immunological disorders with autoimmunity and haemophagocytosis-lymphohistiocytosis. Neurological damage has also been reported due to secondary impairment of the urea cycle [1,2,3]. The disease appears at the time of dietary diversification. It progresses with age and may be discovered in adulthood. There is considerable clinical heterogeneity, with some patients developing severe symptoms of the disease and others showing only mild symptoms.Biologically, the diagnosis is based on the demonstration of hyperammonaemia associated with hyperaminoaciduria and orotic aciduria [4,5]. Lysine, arginine and ornithine are excreted in the urine in excess, while their plasma concentrations are reduced. Arginine and ornithine deficiency alters the function of the urea cycle, leading to hyperammonia following protein ingestion [3]. The treatment of IPD consists of dietary protein restriction and supplementation. into Citrulline, which is well absorbed and efficiently used, so that it partially restores the function of the urea cycle [6]. The aim of this study was to describe the clinical, diagnostic and therapeutic features of dibasic protein intolerance in the Tunisian population.

II. METHODS

II.1. TYPE, LOCATION AND DURATION OF STUDY :

We conducted a retrospective study of 7 cases of IPD collected in the hereditary metabolic diseases unit of the paediatrics department of La Rabta Hospital over a 25-year period from 1992 to 2017. This unit is the reference unit for the management of HMM in Tunisia.

II.2. POPULATION STUDIED :

II.2.1. Patient recruitment :

We cross-referenced the databases of the paediatrics department and the biochemistry laboratory at La Rabta. As the latter is the reference service for the diagnosis of MHM in Tunisia, our sample was representative of Tunisian patients. However, other patients followed up elsewhere than at La Rabta and confirmed abroad, for example, could not be included.

II.2.2. Inclusion criteria :

This study included all children w i t h   PID whose

The positive diagnosis was based on :

• Clinical signs suggestive of the disease: growth retardation, signs of chronic intoxication, osteoporosis, stigmata of haemophagocytosis-lymphohistiocytosis (HLH).
• And the presence of orotic acid in the urine.

• And/or a drop in dibasic amino acids in the blood (by thin layer chromatography).

•And/or urinary elevation (or leakage) of dibasic amino acids (by gas chromatography coupled with mass spectroscopy).

•And/or confirmation of the diagnosis by molecular biology demonstrating a mutation in the SLC7A7 gene.

It should be noted that we included in this study a patient whose diagnosis of IPD was accepted, but part of her file had been lost and some data were missing.

II.3. STUDY TOOLS :

II.3.1. Data collection :

We drew up a study form in which we collected, from the medical records, the epidemiological characteristics of the patients and their families (in particular their geographical origin, consanguinity and family history of IPD), anamnestic data (in particular age, type of first manifestations, psychomotor development, the existence of an aversion to proteins), data from physical examinations (particularly trophicity, abdominal, neurological, pulmonary and bone examinations), biological examinations (particularly ammonia and chromatography of amino acids and organic acids) and radiological examinations (standard X-rays, bone densitometry (BMD), brain imaging, etc.), as well as treatment modalities and diagnosis.), as well as the treatment and evolutionary aspects of the disease (see appendix 1).

II.3.2. Molecular biology study :

Molecular biology data from five patients with IPD followed at the Paediatrics Department of La Rabta Hospital were collected from a publication of work done at the La Rabta Biochemistry Department by

Esseghir N in 2015[10]. The molecular study was carried out by sequencing the SLC7A7 gene.

II.4. DEFINITIONS :

Haemophagocytosis-lymphohistiocytosis: The diagnosis of HLH is based on the presence of clinical and biological criteria. The validated diagnostic criteria are the Janka criteria of the HLH-2004 paediatric protocol [17] For diagnosis, five out of eight criteria are required among: Fever ($\geq$ 38.5 $\circ$C), splenomegaly, bicytopenia (among haemoglobin < 9 g/dL, platelets < 100 G/L, neutrophils < 1000/mm3), elevated triglycerides (> 3.0 mmol/L) or low fibrinogen (< 1.5 g/dL), high ferritin (> 500 ng/mL), image of haemophagocytosis, reduced NK cell cytotoxicity, high soluble CD-25 level (> 2400 IU/mL) [33].

BMD Z-score: The z-score is defined by the standard deviation compared with a population of the same age, and is used to define osteoporosis mainly in children and young adults who have not yet reached peak bone mass. A low Z-score (< - 2) reflects bone loss greater than that usually observed for a given age. Osteopenia is an intermediate stage between normal bones and osteoporosis [34].

Staturo-ponderal retardation: RSP is considered to exist when height is less than 2 standard deviations (SD) from the mean for the child's age and sex, or when there is statural inflection, i.e. a break or progressive inflection in the child's growth curve, or when the child's statural curve is much lower than what is expected for family heights, i.e. less than 2 SD from the corrected target height [35].

Psychomotor delay: this is defined as failure to acquire developmental norms at the programmed ages. Psychomotor delay may be global (affecting all types of acquisition), or concern only one of them [36].

Ammonia: Based on data from the biochemistry laboratory at La Rabta Hospital, normal ammonia is defined as a level of between 0.7 and 55 umol/l.

Bone age: the bone age of our patients was assessed by studying the ossification of the hand and left wrist using the Greulich and Pyle method.

II.5. BIBLIOGRAPHIC RESEARCH :

We collected the literature by consulting the following databases: PubMed, ScienceDirect, EMConsulte.

The keywords used were: "Lysinuric protein intolerance", "macrophage activation", "osteoporosis", "urea cycle", "inherited metabolic disease" .....

Bibliographic references were managed using Endnote X7 software in the Vancouver style, modified to meet the requirements of the Tunis Faculty of Medicine.

II.6. ETHICAL CONSIDERATIONS :

Our study was retrospective. The anonymity of the patients was respected during the writing of the report, and there was no recognisable patient data.

III. RESULTS

III.1. EPIDEMIOLOGICAL CHARACTERISTICS :

Over a 26-year period from 1992 to 2017, seven patients with dibasic protein intolerance were identified.

III.1.1. The distribution of patients b y year of diagnosis :

More than half the cases were diagnosed in the last ten years. Figure 1 shows the distribution of patients by year of diagnosis [Fig 1].

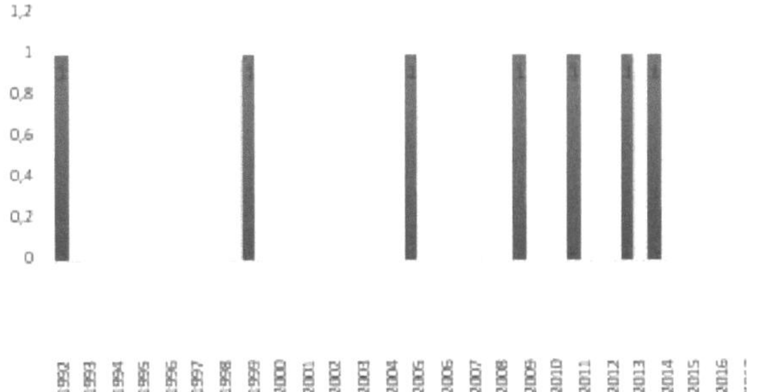

Figure 1: Distribution of patients according to year of diagnosis.

III.1.2. Breakdown of patients in according to of geographical origin :

All our patients came from the west of the country: five from the north-west (Kef = 4, Jendouba = 1) and two from the centre-west (Kasserine = 2) [Fig2].

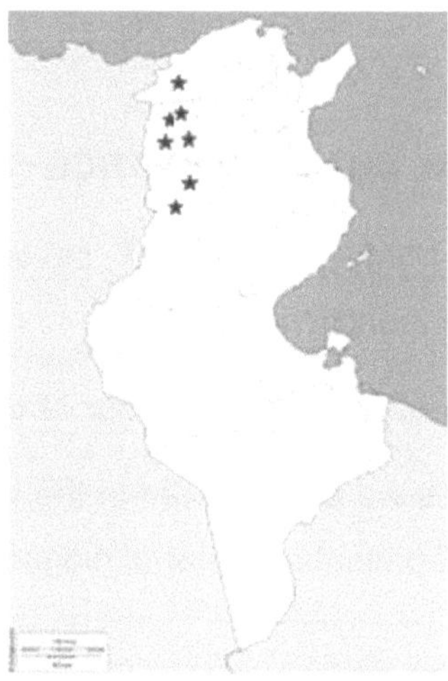

Figure 2:Distribution of patients according to geographical origin.

III.1.3. Distribution of patients according to consanguinity :

Consanguinity was found in all patients. Our patients belonged to five different families. Three of our patients belonged to the same family, including one patient who died at an early age and had another history of death at an early age [Fig 3].

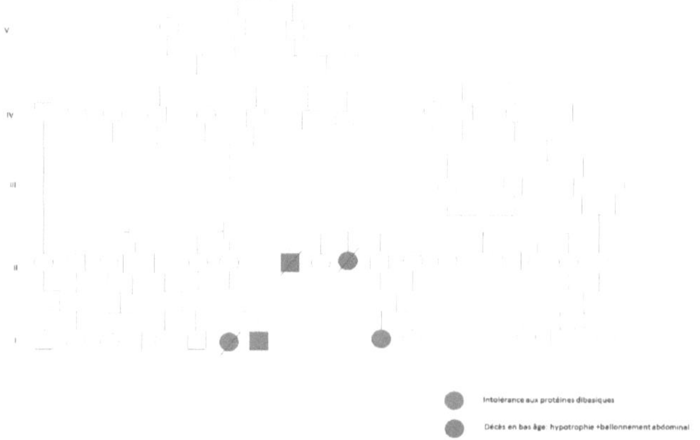

Figure 3: Family tree of patients with IPD.

III.1.4. Breakdown of patients by sex: There was a slight predominance of women, with a sex ratio of 0.4 (five girls and two boys).

III.2. CLINICAL CHARACTERISTICS :

III.2.1. Food diversification :

The median age at diversification was six months [3 - 24 months]. Protein disgust was noted in five patients [Fig 4].

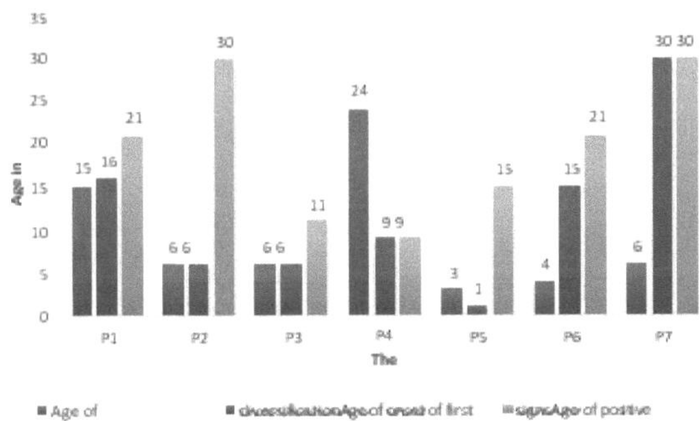

Figure 4: The delay between the age of diversification and the age of positive diagnosis.

III.2.2. Age of first signs :

The age of onset of the first signs in our patients ranged from one day to 16 months, with a median age of nine months [Fig 4].

III.2.3. Diagnosis time :

The median time between the age of diversification and t h e age o f onset of for the first signs of the disease was one month [1 - 24] [Fig 4].

III.2.4. Age of positive diagnosis :

The age of positive diagnosis of the disease ranged from 9 months to 30 months, with a median age of 21 months [Fig 4].

III.2.5. Circumstances of discovery :

RSP associated with hepatosplenomegaly constitute the majority of the revealing signs of the disease, present in almost 70% of patients, followed by abdominal bloating, neurological signs, digestive signs and macrophagic activation syndrome [Fig 5].

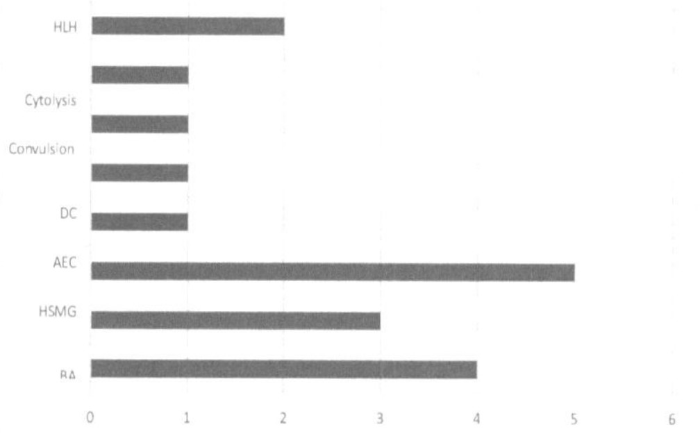

Figure 5: Circumstances of discovery.

RSP: delayed staturo-ponderal; **BA**: abdominal bloating; **HSMG**: hepatosplenomegaly; **AEC**: altered state of health

consciousness; **DC**: chronic diarrhoea; **HLH**: haemophagocytosis-lymphohistiocytosis.

III.2.6. Clinical examination :

Delayed PHN, hepatosplenomegaly and mucocutaneous pallor were present in almost all patients, followed by neurological abnormalities and dyspnoea [Fig 6].

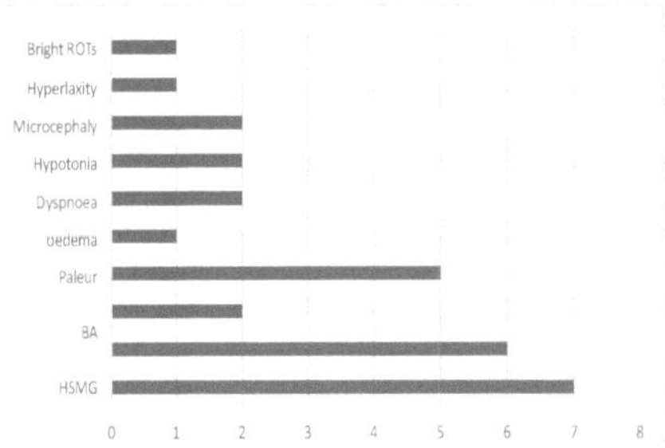

Figure 6: Physical examination data.

III.3. ADDITIONAL EXAMINATIONS :

III.3.1. Data from non-specific additional tests :

III.3.1.1. Biological check-up :

Haematological abnormalities were most frequently found in five patients, in particular biological abnormalities related to HLH in four patients. Hypoalbuminemia was noted in one patient [Fig7].

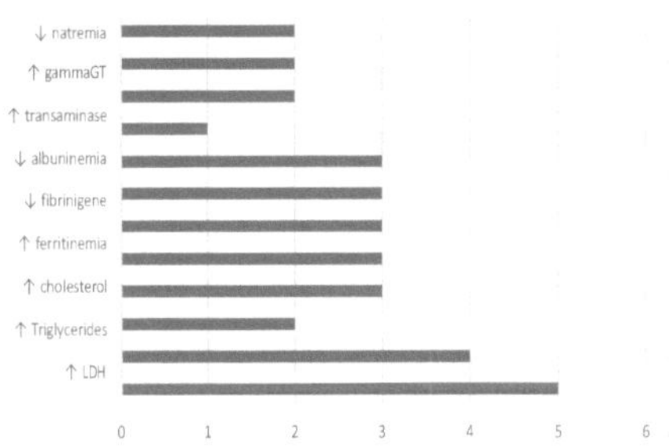

Figure 7: Abnormalities in non-specific biological tests.

↑: Increase↓: Decrease

III.3.1.2. Radiological examination :

Chest X-rays: requested in all patients, had shown an interstitial syndrome in only one patient, but this abnormality was not retained after

11

a chest CT scan was performed.

X-rays of a long bone: requested in three patients, had shown diffuse osteopenia in two patients according to the interpretation mentioned on the reports.

Bone age: requested in five patients, showed a delay in the appearance of ossification points in four patients with AO < AS < AC.

Bone densitometry: performed in four patients, showed osteoporosis in three and was uninterpretable in another because of his young age (4 years). The Z-scores of patients with osteoporosis were -2.4 DS; -4.8 DS and -3.4 DS.

Brain imaging: CT or MRI scans were ordered in patients with neurological signs (n=2) and were normal in both cases.

III.3.1.3. Other investigations :

Myelogram: requested in patients with clinical and laboratory signs of HLH (n=3), it was normal in two cases and showed images of haemophagocytosis in one case.

EEG: requested in the patient who had presented with convulsions, it showed paroxysmal left temporo-occipital anomalies.

EMG: requested in the two patients who had hypotonia on examination and was normal in both patients.

III.3.2. Abnormalities of the specific MHM balance :

III.3.2.1.Hyperammonia :

Ammonia measurements were requested in six patients. Ammonia levels were high in all six cases, with a median level of 112umol/l.

III.3.2.2.Amino acid chromatography :

Amino acid chromatography was of limited value: CAA in blood showed hypoaminoacidaemia in one patient and CAA in urine showed increased secretion of glycine, arginine, alanine and lysine in another.

III.3.2.3.Chromatography of organic acids :

Urine OAC was used for semi-quantitative measurement of orotic acid and showed an increase in orotic acid in all patients, ranging from 7% to 70%.

III.3.3. Molecular biology :

Molecular biology confirmed the positive diagnosis of dibasic protein intolerance. It showed a delTTCT 1471 mutation in the SLCA7A gene in five patients.

Table I: Summary table of signs supporting the diagnosis of IPD.

	P1	P2	P3	P4	P5	P6	P7
Consanguinity	*	*	*	*	*	*	*
Similar cases					*	*	*
Dislike of proteins		*	*	*		*	*
Delayed growth and development	*	*	*	*	*	*	*
Hepatosplenomegaly	*	*	*	*	*	*	
Impaired general condition		*					*
Chronic diarrhoea		*					
Convulsion					*		
Hypotonia	*		*				
Pallor		*	*	*	*	*	
Oedema						*	
Dyspnoea	*				*		
Anemia	*		*	*	*	*	
Leukopenia	*						
Thrombocytopenia			*			*	

Haemophagocytosis-lymphohistiocytosis	*		*	*		*	
↑ lactate dehydrogenase	*		*			*	
↑ triglycerides	*		*			*	
↑ Cholesterol	*		*			*	
↑ Ferritin	*		*	*			
↓ Fibrinogen	*		*	*			
↓Albumin				*		*	
↑ Transaminases			*				
Image of haemophagocytosis				*			
Hyperammonia		*	*	*		*	*
CAA in blood			*				
CAA in urine		*					
↑ Orotic acid	*	*	*	*	*	*	*
SLC7A7 mutation	*	*	*	*		*	
Delayed bone age	*			*	*	*	
Osteopenia			*				*
Osteoporosis				*	*	*	
Fractures						*	*
Psychomotor retardation	*	*		*	*	*	
Hyperammonemic encephalopathy					*		*
Tubulopathy				*	*		

III.4. TREATMENT :

↑: Increase↓: Decrease

III.4.1. The diet :

A hypoprotein diet was prescribed for all patients. Median protein intake was 0.8g/kg/d.

III.4.2. Citrulline :

Citrulline was prescribed for all patients at a median dose of 200 mg/kg/d [100 - 500 mg/kg/d], taken 2 to 3 times a day.

III.5. COMPLICATIONS ARISING FROM THE DISEASE :

III.5.1. Growth abnormalities :

Growth retardation was noted in all our patients, including one case of dwarfism. Height varied between -2.5 DS and -5 DS, with a median height of -3.3 DS.

III.5.2. Nutritional abnormalities :

Protein aversion was noted in five patients. It was associated with undernutrition in three patients, including one with kwashiorkor.

III.5.3. Neurological complications :

Psychomotor delay was noted in five patients, with recovery of psychomotor acquisition under treatment in two patients. One

Hyperammoniemic encephalopathy was observed in two patients following a change in diet and cessation of citrulline treatment in both. In the first patient, the symptomatology consisted of convulsions and behavioural disturbances, with hyperammoniemia of 253 umol/l. The other patient presented with torpor, screaming and abnormal movements with an ammonia level of 73 umol/l.

III.5.4. Skeletal complications :

Two patients had osteopenia complicated in one case by a left supra condylar fracture at the age of 4 years. Three other patients had developed osteoporosis confirmed by BMD, one of which was complicated by multiple fractures (right knee at the age of 1 year and 6 months, right tibia at the age of 3? years, left femur at the age of 5 years). The Z-scores for patients with osteoporosis were -2.4 DS, -4.8 DS and -3.4 DS.

All our patients were given calcium and vitamin D supplements. The three patients with osteoporosis were treated with sodium pamidronate (Aredia$^{®}$) with a number of courses ranging from 3 to 5 depending on the availability of the product and doses ranging from 0.5 to 1 mg/kg/day. Progression on this treatment was marked by an improvement in osteoporosis in only one case, the patient who received 5 courses, with a reduction in Z-score from -4.8 DS at the age of 7.5 years to -3.6 DS at the age of 9 years.

III.5.5. Haematological complications :

Anemia was observed in five patients. This anemia was associated with febrile leuko-neutropenia in one patient and minimal thrombocytopenia ($>100,000e/mm^{3}$) in two patients. Haemophagocytosis-lymphohistiocytosis was observed in four patients. Among these HLH, one The patient had relapsed with this syndrome on three occasions at the ages of 1 year, 2 years and 4 months and 8 years, after which we retained the diagnosis of chronic HLH. The criteria for the diagnosis of HLH are summarised in Table II [Tab II]. All HLH observed were not associated with fever.

Fever	Bicytopenia	SMG	↓Nile	↑ferritinemia	↓fibrinogen	↑TG	LDH	Marrow
P1	*	*		*		*	*	
P2								
P3	*	*	*	*	*	*	*	
P4	*	*		*	*			*
P5								
P6	*	*		*	*	*	*	
P7								

↑: Increase↓: Decrease

Anemia required transfusion of packed red blood cells in two patients, one of whom received 11 transfusions before his haemoglobin levels returned to normal. Febrile neutropenia was treated with dual antibiotic therapy (3ème generation cephalosporin + aminoside). The thrombocytopenia observed did not require platelet transfusion. None of the four patients with haemophagocytosis-lymphohistiocytosis required specific treatment other than IPD.

III.5.6. Renal complications :

Tubulopathy was observed in two patients with polyuria and hypercalciuria. The latter was responsible for bilateral grade I nephrocalcinosis in one patient. In one case, these abnormalities were secondary to treatment with Un alpha. Discontinuation of the treatment led to normalisation of the work-up.

III.5.7. Infectious complications :

We have not noted in this work the existence of recurrent infections or severe sepsis.

III.5.8. Pulmonary complications :

No pulmonary complications were observed in any of our patients.

III.6. EVOLUTION :

III.6.1. Hindsight:

We have a median follow-up of 10.4 years [3 years to 19 and a half years].

III.6.2. Survival :

Six of our patients are currently alive, while one died at the age of three with acute hyperammonemic encephalopathy.

III.6.3. The current state of patients :

From a growth point of view, only two patients caught up with their delayed statural and weight growth. The other five remained behind in terms of height, with height varying between -3.3 and -5 DS, and weight, with P/PMT varying between 75 and 79%. In terms of psychomotor development, only two patients caught up. Three children did not attend school, one of them because of dyslexia. Of the children who did attend school (n=3), only two performed well. Neurologically, two patients retained peripheral hypotonia and another developed epilepsy. The patient with recurrent pathological fractures is currently suffering from immobilisation due to bone pain. As regards the patients with HLH (n=4), we noted a favourable evolution in three of these patients who had normalised their biological anomalies, but they still had hepatosplenomegaly. The fourth patient with HLH had relapsed with this syndrome on three occasions at the ages of 1 year, 2 years and 4 months. and 8 years of age, he continues to have hepatosplenomegaly, elevated ferritin levels, hypofibrinemia and an elevated LDH level suggestive of chronic HLH.

IV. DISCUSSION

IV.1. EPIDEMIOLOGY:

PDI is a disease of unknown prevalence worldwide. In this study, we identified seven cases of IPD over a period of 26 years. First described by Perheetupa and Visakorpi in 1965, PDI has been reported worldwide [7]. Its prevalence is highest in Finland, reaching 1/60,000. To date, patients with non-Finnish PDI have been reported from 24 different countries around the world: mainly documented in Japan, Turkey, Italy and North Africa [4,5,8,9]. In Mauhin's work, sixteen patients with IPD were recorded from 1977 to 2015, which testifies to the rarity of the disease. Five different geographical origins were found: Maghreb (n = 4), France (n = 2), Turkey (n = 1), Lebanon (n = 1) and Guinea (n = 1) [11]. Five Tunisian patients (four families) have already been described [10]. As is often the case with autosomal recessive diseases, consanguinity was found in all our patients, who belonged to five different families. For Mauhin, consanguinity was known for 12/16 patients (9 families, 12 men, 4 women). He did not show any notable personal history, as is the case in our study [11]. Concerning the geographical distribution of patients, we noted that all our patients were from the north-west of the country. This could be explained by a recruitment bias given that our centre is located in the north of the country. The median age of our patients at the time of diagnosis was 21 months, whereas in the literature the median age was 4.1 years (standard deviation: 5.3 years) [11]. The crescendo in the number of cases over the last ten years shows that people are more aware of the need for diagnosis, especially after the Tunisian Association for the Study of Hereditary Metabolic Diseases (ATEMMH) raised doctors' awareness of this rare disease.

IV.2. CLINICAL STUDY :

The median delay between the age of diversification and the onset of the first signs in our patients was 1 month. IPD is a multi-systemic disorder whose clinical onset is usually delayed by breastfeeding or by the use of milk-based infant formulas due to their relatively low protein content. The classic symptoms of IPD may go unnoticed during the first and second decades of life due to subconscious avoidance of dietary protein [12], which explains the median delay between the age of diversification and confirmation of the diagnosis of 6 months, with the longest delay being 30 months.The clinical signs revealing the disease in this study were dominated by delayed height and weight and the presence of hepatosplenomegaly. Neurological and digestive disorders were less common, occurring in two cases each. Since the disease was first described, a great deal of clinical heterogeneity has been observed in patients. IPD is often revealed by the onset of recurrent vomiting and episodes of diarrhoea, poor nutrition, aversion to protein-rich foods, weight stagnation and hepatosplenomegaly [4]. Over time, the clinical picture includes: growth retardation, osteoporosis, pulmonary manifestations (progressive interstitial damage, alveolar proteinosis), renal manifestations (glomerular damage, proximal tubulopathy), haematological manifestations (normochromic or hypochromic anaemia, leucopenia, thrombocytopenia, haemophagocytosis) and a clinical presentation resembling lymphohistiocytosis. Hypercholesterolaemia, hypertriglyceridaemia and acute pancreatitis may also be observed [4, 5, 12]. Muscle hypotonia is observed as early as early childhood. Delayed skeletal maturation is common after the first year of life. Osteoporosis can lead to pathological fractures [12]. In our study, growth retardation and hepatosplenomegaly were consistently found. Blood line abnormalities and bone mineralisation abnormalities were also frequent and present in five patients. Haemophagocytosis lymphohistiocytosis was fairly frequent, documented in four patients, as were lipid balance abnormalities. More rarely, signs in favour of renal involvement were found in two patients, while no cases of pulmonary involvement were found in this series.Neurological signs were frequent in our study, with psychomotor retardation noted in five patients, followed by hypotonia, microcephaly and altered consciousness in the context of hyperamonemic encephalopathy in two patients each. This could be explained by the long delay between the onset of symptoms and the positive diagnosis, as well as deviations from the diet and discontinuation of treatment in some patients. Forced feeding, particularly with protein-rich food, can cause neurological signs with episodes of coma and psychic disorders; this clinical presentation raises suspicions of acute metabolic disorders such as energy deficits in the urea cycle. In fact, the low availability of arginine and ornithine in hepatocytes causes dysfunction of the urea cycle leading to hyperammonemia with hyperammonemic encephalopathy [3]. Here, we briefly discuss some troubling clinical aspects of IPD, emphasising the dichotomy of this disorder: on the one hand, a classic metabolic disease, similar to a moderate urea cycle defect, which may not be difficult to treat; on the other hand, a severe multi-organ disorder in which the therapeutic approach remains difficult [4]. The presence of hepatosplenomegaly may reinforce the suspicion of this metabolic disease. This was found in almost all patients in Sebastio's series [4]. The natural history of this disease can be extremely variable and may not correlate with the nature of the mutations in the SLC7A7 gene, ethnic origin, age of diagnosis or timing of treatment. IPD may be seen in adults with minimal clinical symptoms despite the presence of large gene deletions, as seen in some Italian patients, or it may be diagnosed in very young patients with severe life-threatening disease. In addition, there can be great variation in clinical presentation between individuals sharing the same mutation, as seen in Finland, or even between members of the same family [3].

IV.3. POSITIVE DIAGNOSIS :

Although signs suggestive of IPD were present, diagnosis was delayed (median delay 14.6 months) due to the difficulty of associating non-specific signs with a rare, unrecognised disease. Clinical presentation can vary considerably, and there is no single biochemical study that can easily confirm or exclude the diagnosis. In fact, some patients were suspected of having coeliac disease before the diagnosis was made. Regarding the contribution of the metabolic work-up: hyperammonemia was frequent but not constant, elevated in five patients, whereas CAA was only marginally contributory given the semi-quantitative technique: CAA in the blood showed hypo-aminoacidemia in only one patient and CAA in the urine showed an increase in the secretion of amino acids in another patient. OAC, on the other hand, was contributory, showing an increase in orotic acid in all patients. It is crucial to correlate laboratory results with nutritional status, as biochemical data may be much less informative in malnourished patients. In such cases, it may be necessary to measure renal clearances of dibasic amino acids under the best possible nutritional conditions without exposing the patient to the risk of hyperammonemia [13].

A large amount of additional laboratory data can reinforce the suspicion of a diagnosis of IPD. These include evaluation of complete blood counts and serum protein levels. Myelograms should be limited to cases where there is clinical and biological suspicion of HLH. Osteoporosis, delayed bone age and, most importantly, lung involvement may be seen on X-ray. Abnormal renal function accompanied by proteinuria and haematuria may be present at the time of diagnosis and should be monitored over time [13]. In doubtful cases, it is best to complete the genetic study in search of a disease-specific mutation, which was found in five of our patients, all of whom showed the 1471 delTTCT mutation, which appears to be the mutation found in the Tunisian population [10]. This delTTCT 1471 mutation is one of the 51 SLCA7A-specific mutations identified in 142 patients with IPD [14]. Esseghir et al reported the first prenatal diagnosis by direct mutational analysis of IPD in a Tunisian family showing the same mutation in the homozygous state [15].

Therefore, in all patients with :

-Digestive signs (diarrhoea, vomiting)

-Delayed height and weight

-Osteopenia

$^+$ -/-hypotonia, psychomotor retardation

☐ A work-up should be carried out to look for signs of HLH, which are almost constant from the neonatal period onwards. If this work-up is positive, there is a strong suspicion of IPD and the metabolic work-up should be completed. There should be no hesitation in sending quantitative AAC and molecular biology abroad in cases of strong suspicion (currently not available in Tunisia), but in this case there is the problem of cost abroad.

IV.4. TREATMENT :

All our patients were placed on a hypoprotein diet with citrulline supplementation. None of our patients had received supplementation with other amino acids due to lack of availability. Given the dichotomy of the clinical picture of IPD, there are two main parallel directions of therapy. The first, using a classical metabolic approach, aims to reduce the risk of hyperammoniemia and nutritional supplementation, while the second aims to prevent and treat severe complications [4]. A low-protein diet, which usually requires 0.8-1.5 g protein/kg /day in children and lower amounts (per kg of body weight) in adults, is the mainstay of treatment [4]. Urinary orotic acid can be used as a tool to monitor protein tolerance and urea cycle function. Citrulline supplementation is crucial to treat, at least partially, arginine deficiency through intracellular citrulline metabolism. As previously mentioned, this occurs mainly in the kidney through the action of argininosuccinate synthase, a step which requires aspartate and argininosuccinate lyase. The dosage of L-citrulline was a controversial subject due to the possibility that it could increase damage to the kidney. by its conversion into arginine and NO. L-Citrulline supplementation is therefore generally limited to 100mg/kg/day [4,5]. However, it has been shown that arginine and NO are actually lacking in macrophages and that low plasma concentrations of arginine may be associated with cardiovascular disease. Consequently, the dose may need to be reassessed. A diet restricted in long-chain fatty acids and supplemented with medium-chain fatty acids is also debatable, in order to reduce triglyceride levels and prevent the risk of pancreatitis. Sodium benzoate (100-250 mg/kg/day) may help reduce the risk of hyperammoniemic crisis [4]. Hypocarnitinaemia, which may be present in patients with IPD, is strongly correlated with renal failure, a low-protein diet and the use of ammonia-containing drugs. L-carnitine is therefore supplemented at 25-50 mg/kg/day after measurement of plasma carnitine levels. L-lysine deficiency can be partially corrected by adding low doses of L-lysine (10-40 mg/kg/day orally), although it is not yet known how much can be absorbed [4, 5].

IV.5. COMPLICATIONS OF THE DISEASE :

IV.5.1. Growth abnormalities :

Growth retardation was noted in all our patients. No growth hormone deficiency was observed in any of the four patients evaluated, and none of them had received growth hormone injections. This delay is generally observed in children with IPD and is generally related to protein malnutrition [16]. In some cases, growth hormone deficiency or arginine depletion leading to impaired growth hormone secretion has been observed [16]. Growth hormone has been used in several individuals with a good response [16]. All patients of Muhin et al (16/16) presented with growth failure at a mean age of 2 years (standard deviation: 3.6 years). Growth hormone improved height in 2/2 patients who presented with concomitant GH deficiency. Among the 11 patients with available data, the last available mean height was -2.51 SD [11].

IV.5.2. Digestive and nutritional complications :

A dislike of protein was noted in five of our patients. In Mauhin, aversion to protein-rich food was observed in nine out of 16 patients, with associated diarrhoea and vomiting, leading to continuous enteral nutrition in four patients and parenteral nutrition in three others [11]. Increased plasma concentrations of cholesterol and triglycerides, found in three of our patients, are relatively common in people with IPD [17]. In these patients, these lipid abnormalities were part of the biological disturbances associated with HLH. For Tanner et al, these lipid balance disturbances were observed outside of HLH. No clear explanation has been proposed for this dyslipidaemic state; a carbohydrate-rich diet may contribute to the increase in plasma triglyceride concentration, but it is not sufficient to explain hypercholesterolaemia or severe hypertriglyceridaemia (triglycerides > 1000 mg/dL or > 11 mmol/L).

Finally, several other deficiencies were also observed, such as hypocarnitinaemia (3 cases) and low plasma selenium concentrations (in 4 of the 5 cases examined) [11]. These tests were not performed in our patients.

IV.5.3. Neurological complications :

Neurological complications were fairly frequent in this series, with various manifestations: hypotonia, convulsions, psychomotor retardation and acute hyperamoniac encephalopathy. In the literature, intellectual development is usually normal unless episodes of prolonged coma cause neurological damage, according to Nunes [12]. A secondary disorder of the urea cycle with hyperammoniaemia has been well described in IPD. Indeed, it is thought that low arginine and ornithine levels lead primarily to functional depletion of urea cycle intermediates. However, more than half of the patients described by Palacin et al had cognitive problems that can easily be explained by chronic hyperammonia [18]. As far as chronic dyslipidaemia is concerned, no case of stroke has been reported. In the study by Mauhin [11], five out of 16 patients presented with acute hyperammoniemic encephalopathy, with convulsions in four patients and coma in three. Persistent hypotonia and impaired psychomotor development were recorded in eight patients with no significant association with elevated glutamine levels. Another patient presented with convulsive seizures due to a complicated cholesteatoma. In acute hyperammoniemic crises, treatment consists of intravenous administration of arginine chloride and nitrogen-containing drugs (sodium benzoate, sodium phenylacetate) to block ammonia production, combined with reduction of excess nitrogen in the diet by providing energy in the form of carbohydrates to reduce catabolism [12].

IV.5.4. Skeletal complications :

Five of our patients had abnormalities in bone mineralisation, with two cases of osteopenia, three cases of osteoporosis and two cases of multiple pathological fractures. In Parto's work, although the criteria for osteopenia were limited to bone radiography, osteopenia was reported in the majority of patients. He also described histological signs of osteoporosis in 8 out of 9 patients [19]. Collagen synthesis in skin fibroblasts was decreased. The mechanism involved in the development of osteopenia seems to be more associated with synthesis defects secondary to protein depletion than with increased degradation by osteoclasts or inflammation [19]. A case series reported 6 Turkish patients with IPD (age range: 11 to 36 years) who had bone mineral density Z-scores ranging from -2.1 to -5.8 [20]. Similarly, in a cohort of 9 Italian patients, 2 patients had osteoporosis [20]. In a study of 29 Finnish patients (aged 3.7 to 47.9 years), 13 showed radiographic signs of osteoporosis [21]. Fifty-seven fractures were reported in 20 of these patients, with the number of fractures per patient ranging from 0 to 7 [19,21]. Most fractures occurred before the age of 15 and were associated with minor trauma [21]. Interestingly, fractures occurred as frequently in patients with osteoporosis as in patients without radiological evidence of osteoporosis [19,21].

The efficacy of the recommended treatment to improve osteoporosis in IPD remains unclear. A 2-year study of 19 patients (1.9 to 32.7 years) treated with citrulline with or without lysine supplementation did not improve osteoporosis [22]. There is a single report of the use of alendronate in an 11-year-old girl with LPI, with an improvement in bone density after one year of treatment [24]. Zoledronic acid was started in the Posay patient before his diagnosis of IPD, and during the first year of treatment, the frequency of fracture decreased [23].

Our three patients with osteoporosis were started on sodium pamidronate. Only in one case, the patient who received 5 courses of treatment, did the osteoporosis improve from a Z-score of -4.8 DS at the age of 7.5 years to -3.6 DS at the age of 9 years.

IV.5.5. Haematological and infectious complications :

Blood line abnormalities were common, observed in five of our patients. The most frequent abnormality was anaemia, followed by thrombocytopenia and, more rarely, leuko-neutropenia. In the literature, haematological abnormalities are frequently observed in the mild form of normochromic or hypochromic anaemia, leucopenia and thrombocytopenia [20]. These abnormalities generally do not cause any clinical symptoms unless they progress to the clinical picture of HLH observed on several occasions in IPD [25,26]. HLH was considered in four patients, one of whom had presented with chronic HLH. The criteria for HLH consistently found were bicytopenia, splenomegaly and elevated ferritinemia. Fever was absent in all our patients and haemophagocytosis was seen in only one patient, whereas in the literature, patients with IPD have fever with haemophagocytosis in the bone marrow and laboratory abnormalities identical to those seen in other forms of HLH [25,26]. None of our patients had received any specific treatment for HLH other than IPD. In Mauhin's work, specific treatment of HLH was necessary for two patients. Both received corticosteroids and cyclosporine, which was effective in only one case [11]. Indeed, treatment with cyclosporine A, corticosteroids and intravenous immunoglobulin have been tried with some success, but a definite therapeutic approach has not been established. Three of our patients had a favourable outcome, while another had relapsed three times before becoming chronic. The indication for treatment in the latter patient remains debatable. However, we did not note any serious or recurrent infections.

Other pathologies reflecting an altered immune response in IPD that have been observed in the literature but not reported in our patients include: systemic lupus erythematosus, vasculitis, severe generalised varicella and EBV infection, impaired lymphocyte and mildly deficient B-cell function, hypergammaglobulinaemia or low serum immunoglobulin concentrations and hypocomplementaemia [12].

IV.5.6. Renal complications :

We noted stigmata of tubulopathy such as polyuria and hypercalciuria in two patients. In one case, these abnormalities were iatrogenic, secondary to treatment with Un alpha. Discontinuation of treatment resolved these abnormalities. With regard to renal impairment in IPD, proteinuria and microscopic haematuria are frequent urine sediment abnormalities. Isolated mild proteinuria is the initial sign of renal disease leading to proximal tubular dysfunction and nephrocalcinosis [11,27]. Membranous or mesangial glomerulonephritis and Fanconi syndrome have been reported in several patients, but data on long-term renal prognosis were scarce. Renal tubular acidosis or findings consistent with reduced phosphate reabsorption and generalised aminoaciduria indicate underlying complex proximal tubular disease (Fanconi). Renal histology reveals immune-mediated glomerulonephritis and chronic tubulointerstitial nephritis with glomerulosclerosis in the absence of immune deposits [27]. In Tanner's study, proteinuria and haematuria were observed in 74% and 38% of patients respectively. Mean serum creatinine and cystatin C concentrations were increased in 38% and 59% of patients respectively. Elevated blood pressure was present in 36% of patients, four of whom (10.2%) developed end-stage renal disease requiring dialysis, and 59% developed mild to moderate renal failure [28]. There were no specific histological findings in the renal biopsy. Non-specific chronic tubulo-interstitial lesions are the most common and may be associated with nephrocalcinosis secondary to hypercalciuria [29]. Glomerular lesions are more variable and unpredictable: lupus-like lesions and amyloidosis may be observed. Therefore, renal biopsy should be reserved for patients with glomerular symptoms in order to adjust treatment and follow-up. These impressive data indicate that kidney damage is a serious and frequent complication that requires careful and constant assessment. The pathogenesis of renal damage is unknown but may be associated with overproduction of nitric oxide [29].

IV.5.7. Pulmonary complications :

There were no cases of pulmonary involvement in our series. In IPD, progressive interstitial changes in the lungs are frequently detected in the early years without overt clinical symptoms. Progression to severe pulmonary alveolar proteinosis (PAP) is a well-known life-threatening complication, occurring as early as childhood in many people w i t h IPD [11]. Fibrosispulmonary disease can also develop independently of PAP. Lung involvement begins as an asymptomatic interstitial disease that can be diagnosed by conventional chest X-ray. The mechanism leading to lung damage or its progression is not clear. It may be associated with an accumulation of intracellular nitric oxide [11]. Progression is marked by the appearance of reticulo-nodular interstitial densities visible on chest X-rays and better assessed by high-resolution chest CT, which shows ground-glass opacities with superimposed smooth septal thickening [30]. PAP usually presents with progressive exertional dyspnoea, tachypnoea and cough exacerbated by respiratory infections and complicated by viral or bacterial pneumonia. Signs of struggle, cyanosis and, more rarely, hippocratic features may be found on physical examination. At this stage, bronchoalveolar lavage may demonstrate that the airspace is invaded by increased numbers of foamy cells and macrophages filled with proteinaceous material suggestive of alveolar proteinosis [19]. Attempts to control this potentially fatal complication include the use of high-dose corticosteroids and the administration of granulocyte-macrophage colony-stimulating factor with very limited success. The most effective tool for controlling the progression of alveolar proteinosis is complete lung lavage [31]. A heart-lung transplant controlled the respiratory status of a young Italian patient for 18 months, before EBV infection triggered progressive respiratory failure and death [32].

IV.6. THE PROGNOSIS OF THE DISEASE :

With a median follow-up of 10.4 years, six of our patients are currently alive. One patient died at the age of three with acute hyperammoniac encephalopathy following a change in diet and cessation of citrulline treatment. The prognosis of IPD is variable, depending mainly on pulmonary complications, which we did not observe in our patients and which constitute a poor prognostic factor and the main cause of death from this disease. In the literature, Parenti et al report, in their series of 9 Italian patients, three deaths at the age of 6 ½, 10 ½ and 11 years, one of which in a context of respiratory superinfection, with, on histological analysis of the lung at autopsy, a PAP. The causes of death of the other two patients are not known [20]. Cases of early death were also reported by Parto et al [19]. There were four deaths secondary to respiratory failure in children under 15 years of age, diagnosed on average at 5.8 years of age and dying at 10, 13, 7 and 3 years of age. Similarly, in the work by Mauhin [11], six patients presented with pulmonary involvement (mean age at diagnosis: 2.24 years). They all died of respiratory failure at a mean age of 4.0 years. Mauhin et al had also shown that younger age at diagnosis was a borderline predictor of shorter survival (p = 0.16) [11]. Bivariate prediction of survival by age-adjusted plasma lysine levels and age at diagnosis suggests that their influence on prognosis is independent and additive (p = 0.10) [11]. Patients with PAP had a non-significant trend towards higher plasma lysine levels than those without PAP (p = 0.11) [11]. The potential association between intellectual disability and time of diagnosis was assessed in 32 patients with IPD. Those diagnosed before the age of 5 (n = 16) were significantly more likely (P = 0.03) to have an intellectual disability than those diagnosed at an older age [37]. Similarly, patients diagnosed earlier had a lower incidence of intellectual disability [37].

V.CONCLUSIONS

Dibasic protein intolerance or protein intolerance with lysinuria (PTI) is an autosomal recessive inherited metabolic disorder. It is linked to a defect in the membrane transport of the dibasic amino acids Arginine, Ornithine and Lysine caused by a mutation in the SLC7A7 gene encoding the y + LAT-1 subunit of the transmembrane transporter of dibasic amino acids. This transporter is expressed in the basolateral membrane of the renal tubule, the cells of the intestine, the lung, the spleen and in circulating monocytes and macrophages, which would explain the broad spectrum of symptoms described, These include growth retardation, protein intolerance, hepatosplenomegaly, osteoporosis, pulmonary involvement, renal failure, immunological disorders with autoimmunity and haemophagocytosis-lymphohistiocytosis. Neurological damage has also been reported due to the secondary disorder of the urea cycle. The aim of this study was to describe the clinical, diagnostic and therapeutic features of dibasic protein intolerance in Tunisia. We conducted a retrospective study in the hereditary metabolic diseases unit of the paediatric department of Hôpital la Rabta over a 26-year period from 1992 to 2017. Inclusion criteria were patients with clinical signs compatible with IPD associated with orotic aciduria on organic acid chromatography. We identified 7 patients with IPD. Among them, five werefrom the north-west of the country and the other two from the centre-west. All our patients had consanguineous parents. Three of them were related. Despite the autosomal recessive nature of the disease, we observed a predominance of females, with a sex ratio of 0.4. The median age of onset was 9 months [1 day-16 months], with a median delay after feeding of 1 month [1- 30 months]. The median age at diagnosis was 21 months [9-30 months].The clinical manifestations of the disease were variable. Growth retardation (n=7) and hepatosplenomegaly (n=6) were almost constant signs of the disease, followed by protein aversion (n=5), pallor associated with anaemia (n=5) and neurological signs (n=4) such as convulsions, altered consciousness, hypotonia and microcephaly. Digestive signs were infrequent, with chronic diarrhoea noted in only one patient.

Blood count abnormalities were frequent, affecting all three blood lines. This disorder was associated with other clinical and laboratory signs, leading to the diagnosis of haemophagocytosis-lymphohistiocytosis in four patients. Lipid disturbances such as hypercholesterolaemia and hypertriglyceridaemia were observed in two patients. Hypoalbuminemia was noted in only one patient. Radiological findings included delayed bone age in four patients, osteoporosis in three and osteopenia in two.

Ammonia was elevated in 6 patients, with a median of 112umol/l. Amino acid chromatography was of limited value, being informative in only one case each: one hypoaminoacidaemia in one patient and urinary leakage of dibasic amino acids in another.The positive diagnosis was confirmed by molecular biology in five patients, which showed the delTTCT 1471 mutation in the SLCA7A gene in these patients.A low-protein diet and citrulline supplementation in doses ranging from 100 to 500 mg/kg/day were prescribed for all our patients.Despite treatment, complications were observed in our patients. Growth retardation was noted in all our patients, with dwarfism (height = -5 DS) in one of them. Neurological complications were frequent, such as slowing of psychomotor development (n=5) and acute hyperammonemic encephalopathy following a change in diet or cessation of citrulline treatment (n=2). The anaemia observed in five patients required transfusion with packed red blood cells in two, one of whom received 11 transfusions before his haemoglobin levels returned to normal. All anaemic patients were treated with martial therapy and folic acid supplementation. None of the four patients with haemophagocytosis-lymphohistiocytosis required any specific treatment apart from IPD. Bone involvement was complicated by pathological fractures in two cases. The Z-scores of patients with osteoporosis (n=3) were -2.4 DS, -4.8 DS and -3.4 DS. They were started on pamidronate sodium (Aredia®) with a number of courses ranging from three to five and doses ranging from 0.5 to 1 mg/kg/d. Only the patient who received five courses showed improvement in osteoporosis. Renal damage with stigmata of tubulopathy was noted in two patients. No recurrent infections or pulmonary involvement were noted.After a median follow-up of 11 years [3 years - 19 and a half years], six of our patients are currently alive. One patient died at the age of three with acute hyperammoniac encephalopathy. Five patients have retained growth retardation. Two patients caught up with their psychomotor development. They attended school with good academic performance, whereas three others did not attend school because of dyslexia. Two patients retained peripheral hypotonia and four retained hepatosplenomegaly, one of which was associated with chronic macrophagic activation syndrome.

Our study was open to criticism because of its limitations: the small sample size, explained by the rarity of the disease, but also by a possible recruitment bias, since we did not take into account any patients diagnosed and followed up in other departments, this work not being a multicentre study, and the lack of certain data given its retrospective nature. Despite these limitations, this study remains interesting. Indeed, despite its small size, the number of our patients is comparable to that of other series, and only the Finnish series reported a larger number. The long follow-up period gave us a better idea of the complications and long-term evolution of the disease. Finally, it enabled us to achieve our objectives:

– A description of the clinical features of the disease, which will give a better understanding of the disease and encourage people to suspect it, especially when faced with a clinical picture of delayed growth and hepatosplenomegaly associated with neurological manifestations beginning after the age of diversification.

– Emphasise the difficulties of positive diagnosis in the absence of specific biochemical analysis of the disease, with amino acid chromatography contributing little. We suggest that molecular biology should be used for confirmation, as this is currently possible in Tunisia. Molecular biology enabled us to identify a mutation that is common in Tunisia.

– Emphasising the limitations of the treatment available makes it difficult to manage the disease and, above all, its complications, and means that regular, long-term monitoring is essential.

REFERENCES

[1] Torrents D, Mykkänen J, Pineda M, Feliubadaló L, Estévez R, de Cid R et al. Identification of SLC7A7, encoding y + LAT-1, as the lysinuric protein intolerance gene. Nat Genet. 1999;21:293-6.

[2] Borsani G, Bassi MT, Sperandeo MP, De Grandi A, Buoninconti A, Riboni M et al. SLC7A7, encoding a putative permease-related protein, is mutated in patients with lysinuric protein intolerance. Nat Genet. 1999;21:297-301.

[3] Simell 0, Striver CR, Beaudet AL, Sly WS, Vailc D. The Merobolic Basis of Inherited Disease. New York: McGraw Hill; 1989.

[4] Sebastio G, Sperandeo MP, Andria G. Lysinuric protein intolerance: reviewing concepts on a multisystem disease. Am J Med Genet. 2011;157:54-62.

[5] Ogier H, Schiff M, Dionisi-Vici C. Lysinuric protein intolerance (LPI): A multi organ disease by far more complex than a classic urea cycle disorder. Mol Genet Metab. 2012;106:12-7.

[6] Rajantie J, Simell O, Rapola J, Perheentupa J. Lysinuric protein intolerance: a two-year trial of dietary supplementation therapy with citrulline and lysine. J Pediatr. 1980;97:927-32.

[7] Sperandeo MP, Andria G, Sebastio G. Lysinuric protein intolerance: update and extended mutation analysis of the SLC7A7 gene. Hum Mutat. 2008;29:14-21.

[8] Perheentupa J, Visakorpi JK. Protein intolerance with deficient transport of basic amino acids. Another inborn error of metabolism. Lancet. 1965;2:813-6.

[9] Noguchi A, Nakamura K, Murayama K, Yamamoto S, Komatsu H, Kizu R et al. Clinical and genetic features of lysinuric protein intolerance in japan. Pediatr Int. 2016;58(10):979-83.

[10] Esseghir N, Bouchlaka CS, Fredj SH, Ben Chehida A, Azzouz H,

Fontaine M et al. 1471 delTTCT a Common Mutation of Tunisian Patients with Lysinuric Protein Intolerance. Clin Lab. 2015;61(12):1973-7.

[11] Mauhin W, Habarou F, Gobin S, Update on Lysinuric Protein Intolerance, a Multi-faceted Disease Retrospective cohort analysis from birth to adulthood. Orphanet J Rare Dis. 2017;12(1):3.

[12] Nunes V, Niinikoski H. Lysinuric Protein Intolerance [Online]. University of Washington [cited 2006/10/21]; [approximately 33 screens]. Available from URL:https://www.ncbi.nlm.nih.gov/ pubmed/20301535.

[13]Simell O, Scriver CR, Beaudet AL, Sly WS, Valle DT. Lysinuric protein intolerance and other cationic aminoacidurias. J Inherit Metab Dis. 2011;49:334-56.

[14] Font-Llitjos M, Rodriguez-Santiago B, Espino M. Novel SLC7A7 large rearrangements in lysinuric protein intolerance patients involving the same AluY repeat. Eur J Hum Genet. 2009;17:71-9.

[15] Esseghir N, Bouchlaka CS, Fredj SH, Chehida AB, Azzouz H, Fontaine M et al. First report of a molecular prenatal diagnosis in a Tunisian family with lysinuric protein intolerance. JIMD Rep. 2011;1:37-8.

[16]Niinikoski H, Lapatto R, Nuutinen M, Tanner L, Simell O, Nanto-Salonen K. Growth hormone therapy is safe and effective in patients with lysinuric protein intolerance. JIMD Rep. 2011;1:43-7.

[17] Tanner LM, Niinikoski H, Nanto-Salonen K, Simell O. Combined hyperlipidemia in patients with lysinuric protein intolerance. J Inherit Metab Dis. 2010;33Suppl3:S145-S50.

[18] Palaćın M, Bertran J, Chillarón J, Estévez R, Zorzano A. Lysinuric protein intolerance: mechanisms of pathophysiology. Mol Genet Metab. 2004;81Suppl1:S27-S37.

[19]Parto K, Penttinen R, Paronen I, Pelliniemi L, Simell O. Osteoporosis in lysinuric protein intolerance. J Inherit Metab Dis. 1993;16:441-50.

[20]Parenti G, Sebastio G, Strisciuglio P, Incerti B, Pecoraro C,

Terracciano L. Lysinuric protein intolerance characterized by bone marrow abnormalities and severe clinical course, J Pediatr. 1995;126:246-51.

[21]Svedstrom E, Parto K, Marttinen M, Virtama P, Simell O. Skeletal manifestations of lysinuric protein intolerance. A follow-up study of 29 patients. Skelet Radiol. 1993;22:11-6.

[22] Rajantie J, Simell O, Rapola J, Perheentupa J. Lysinuric protein intolerance: a two-year trial of dietary supplementation therapy with citrulline and lysine. J Pediatr. 1980;97:927-932.

[23] Posey JE, Burrage LC, Miller MJ, Liu P, Hardison MT, Elsea SH, et al. Lysinuric Protein Intolerance Presenting with Multiple Fractures. Mol Genet Metab Rep. 2014;1:176-183.

[24] Gomez L, Garcia-Cazorla A, Gutierrez A, Artuch R, Varea V, Martin J et al. Treatment of severe osteoporosis with alendronate in a patient with lysinuric protein intolerance. J Inherit Metab Dis. 2006;29:687.

[25] Doireau V, Fenneteau O, Duval M, Perelman S, Vilmer E, Touati G et al. Lysinuric dibasic protein intolerance: Characteristic aspects of bone marrow involvement. Arch Pediatr. 1996;3:877- 80.

[26] Duval M, Fenneteau O, Doireau V, Faye A, Emilie D, Yotnda P et al. Intermittent hemophagocytic lymphohistiocytosis is a regular feature of lysinuric protein. J Pediatr. 1996;13:236-9.

[27] Estève E, Krug P, Hummel A, Arnoux JB, Boyer O, Brassier A e al. Renal involvement in lysinuric protein intolerance: contribution of pathology to assessment of heterogeneity of renal lesions. Hum Pathol. 2017;62:160-9.

[28] Tanner LM, Nanto-Salonen K, Niinikoski H, Jahnukainen T, Keskinen P, Saha H et al. Nephropathy advancing to end-stage renal disease: A novel complication of lysinuric protein intolerance. Pediatrics. 2007;150:631-4.

[29] Nicolas C, Bednarek N, Vuiblet V, Boyer O, Brassier A, De Lonlay P

et al. Renal Involvement in a French Paediatric Cohort of Patients with Lysinuric Protein Intolerance. JIMD Rep. 2016;29:11- 17.

[30]Santamaria F, Parenti G, Guidi G, Rotondo A, Grillo G, Larocca MR et al. Early detection of lung involvement in lysinuric protein intolerance: Role of high-resolution computed tomography and radioisotopic methods. Am J Respir Crit Care Med. 1996;153:731-5.

[31] Ceruti M, Rodi G, Stella GM, Adami A, Bolongaro A, Baritussio A et al. Successful whole lung lavage in pulmonary alveolar proteinosis secondary to lysinuric protein intolerance: A case report. Orphanet J Rare Dis. 2007;2:14.

[32] Santamaria F, Brancaccio G, Parenti G, Francalanci P, Squitieri C, Sebastio G et al. Recurrent fatal pulmonary alveolar proteinosis after heart-lung transplantation in a child with lysinuric protein intolerance. J Pediatr. 2004;145:268-72.

[33] Henter JI, Horne A, Aricó M, Egeler RM, Filipovich AH, Imashuku S et al. HLH-2004: diagnostic and therapeutic guidelines for hemophagocytic lymphohistiocytosis. Pediatr Blood Cancer. 2007;48:124-31.

[34] Raphaël G, Dan B, Philippe O. APOROSE : Aide à la Prise en Charge de l'Ostéoporose en soins primaires [Online]. Faculté de médecine Paris Diderot, 29/01/2014 [cited 2017/10/03];[about 5 screens]. Available from URL: http://aporose.fr/esp_dmo.php.

[35] Bourillon A, Benoist G, Delacourt C. Normal and pathological growth [Online]. Université Médicale Virtuelle Francophone,01/12/2014 [cited 20/05/2018];[about 15 screens]. Available from URL: http://campus.cerimes.fr/media/campus/deploiement/pediatrie/enseignem ent/croissance_normale/ site/html/1.html.

[36] Bourillon A, Benoist G, Delacourt C. Psychomotor development [Online]. Université Médicale Virtuelle Francophone,01/12/2014 [cited 20/05/2018];[approximately 16 screens]. Available from

URL:http://campus.cerimes.fr/media/campus/deploiement/pediatrie/enseig
nement/developpemen t_psychomoteur/site/html/1.html.

[37] Noguchi A, Nakamura K,Murayama K, Yamamoto S, Komatsu H,
Kizu R et al. Clinical and genetic features of lysinuric protein intolerance
in Japan. Pediatr Int. 2016;58(10):979-983.

Dibasic protein intolerance straddles the line between the metabolic and the autoimmune.

Appendix 1: Data collection form for the IPD.

Dibasic protein intolerance

N° Dossier :

Name:

First name:

Date of birth:

Gender:

Geographical origin:

Consanguinity: yes / no$_1$ st $_D$ 2th $_D$3th$_D$ **Genetic investigation:**

Similar cases

Death in infancy:

Personal history :

Pregnancy:

Giving birth :

Power supply :

Breast milk :

Mixed breastfeeding :

Age of diversification :

DPM:

Smile response:

Seated:

Stand up:

Walking :

Speech:

Cleaning :

School level :

☐ Good DPM / RPM

Age of discovery of the disease:

First event:

Dibasic protein intolerance straddles the line between the metabolic and the autoimmune.

Time to diagnosis:

Clinical signs :

P :

T :

PC :

P/PMT :

BMI :

Curve break: yes /no Fever:/prolonged Neurological examination:

Pleuropulmonary examination

Abdominal examination :

HMG :

SMG :

Osteoarticular examination :

Skin/ muscle/ skin examination

Further examination :

GB :	HG:	PNN :	LC :	Plaq :	Retic :
VGM :	TCMH :				
Vs :	CRP :	ASAT :	ALAT :	gGT :	LDH :
TG :					
CPK :	LDH :	CI :			
IONO :		ferritin :			
GDS :					

Myelogram:

Ammonia :

CAA

Dibasic protein intolerance straddles the line between the metabolic and the autoimmune.

CAD :

Molecular biology :

Bone age :

DMO :

EEG :

EMG :

cMRI :

Radio standards :

Complications :

Growth :

Weight stagnation

Growth retardation

Dwarfism

Food :

Aversion to proteins

malnutrition

Neurological :

RPM

Hypcrammonemic encephalopathy

Coma

Skeletal :

Osteopathy

Osteoporosis

Fractures

Haematological :

Anemia

Thrombocytopenia

Leukopenia

Aplasia

SAMoui /non

Number of criteria

Fever prolonged, bi or pancytopenia,

SMG, hyponatremia, hyperferritinaemia,

hypofebrinemia, hyper triglyceridemia, LDH increase, CD25 increase,
haemophagocytosis image

Dibasic protein intolerance straddles the line between the metabolic and the
autoimmune.

Renal :

- Tubulopathy

- HTA

- NEG

- Nephrotic syndrome

- IRC

Infectious : Sites :
Pulmonary :
- Interstitial lung disease

- Alveolar proteinosis

- Alveolar haemorrhage

Treatment:

☐ Basic treatment:

-citrulline : yes /no

Dose :

Duration:

- Plan

- Lysine supplementation   carnitine

- Oligo E supplementation :

☐ Complications treatment :

- Antibiotic

- Vaccination

- Immunoglobulin

- Corticoides

- GCSF

- Immunosuppressant

- Biphosphanate

- GH

- Alveolar lavage

Step back:

Dibasic protein intolerance straddles the line between the metabolic and the autoimmune.

Evolution:

Current status:

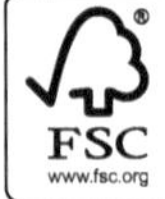

Printed by Books on Demand GmbH, Norderstedt / Germany